Stop
Stopping

Scott Dillon

ISBN: 0-646-97528-5
ISBN-13: 978-0-646-97528-3

DEDICATION

To my Father who taught me to MOVE
To my Mother who taught me to CARE
To Aroha who taught me to LOVE.

CONTENTS

Out of the night that covers me,
Black as the pit from pole to pole,
I thank whatever gods may be
For my unconquerable soul.

In the fell clutch of circumstance
I have not winced nor cried aloud.
Under the bludgeoning of chance
My head is bloody, but unbowed.

Beyond this place of wrath and tears
Looms but the Horror of the shade,
And yet the menace of the years
Finds, and shall find me, unafraid.

It matters not how strait the gate,
How charged with punishments the scroll,
I am the master of my fate:
I am the captain of my soul.

Invictus
BY WILLIAM ERNEST HENLEY

1 INTRODUCTION

"The wound is the place where the Light enters you."
— Jalaluddin Rumi

PHASE ONE - The Break.

I sat on the sand at Greenhills, Cronulla Beach.

It was overcast, cold and raining. I sat there all alone on the first Saturday of winter 2007.

I had been going through this life for 6 years...

Living pay check to pay check. Getting good money relative to other guys my age – only because I was working so many hours.

I was managing truck drivers. I would work from 3am-5pm most weekdays.

Get my paycheck...Then write myself off all weekend.

Drugs.

Alcohol.

With the confidence of a tissue box, the only way I felt I could connect and communicate with others and meet other people was under the cloud of a chaotic cocktail of stimulants and depressants.

Each few months the quantity increased.

Always smiling, and saying everything was 'ok' and that I'm 'good'...

But in that moment, with the rain falling on me, while looking out at the white-caps on the waves, and not a soul around... All of a sudden, the years caught up to me.

I let my head fall into my hands and I cried.

Cried... Like I never cried before.

Whaling... Noises coming out of me that I didn't know existed.

I felt physically empty.

Like an old, rusted bucket, left out in the rain...

That my life had been such a waste, and would never amount to anything.

I asked myself what I could possibly do to change, to feel better...

As the tears continued to pour out of my eyes, I looked up as the rain fell on me. In that moment, I felt as if the world was also, crying on me.

Both our tears blended together...

"This is how it is" I thought.

Disappointed...

Disappointed, that all the stories I was told in school as a kid about how life was meant to be and how it was meant to look like were all untrue.

At least for me.

I had no answers.

So, for the next 30 minutes I contemplated all the ways I could end my life.

I remember doing it with such ease. Just like choosing a meal off a restaurant menu.

Selecting the ones that would impact those around me the least.

"How am I meant to get out of this?"

"I can never change how I feel…"

A man ran by in the rain, laughing with his dog… it did absolutely nothing for how I felt.

It just made me feel worse.

"I WISH I could be that happy…"

"If only I had better friends…"

But who?

"If only I had a better job…"

But doing what?

"If only I had other things to do…"

If only…

If only.

I sat there and looked up.

It was still raining.

But I had no more tears to give.

Hollow, alone, with nothing to lose.

Nothing.

Something came through me.

I decided, like most people, that I would run away from my problems.

I would sell everything I had.

And travel.

So I did.

PHASE TWO - The False Fix.

So here I was.

Masking how I really felt by living a life of adventure.

I was feeling like I was invincible and by not caring if I died, my ego was at an all-time high.

With no experience climbing a mountain at all, I decided I would climb one of the highest mountains in South America.

By 9pm that night I began climbing.

No idea what I was doing. Figuring it out as I went.

...Until 3am the following morning.

At 5,520m above sea level, after climbing for the past 6 hours one of the most severe cases of altitude sickness (HAPE) began to set in.

Vomiting everywhere, my head feeling like it was being crushed by two forceps, hardly able to see, and with absolutely no energy, the only way I would survive was to get back down to basecamp.

With no support except for an unqualified Ecuadorian to help guide me, I was only hours from losing my life.

Not me choosing to make it happen this time, but the universe choosing to make it happen for me.

As I fought for my life—WANTING my life, for the first time, in all my life.

Things were different.

I was not thinking about what I didn't have.

But what I did.

With vomit and blood all over my face I remember looking up at the stars that seemed to be tenfold what I had ever seen in my life.

And felt this overwhelming sense of peace, beauty, one-ness.

I didn't know what there was to live for, but I began to feel something.

PHASE THREE - The Death.

I truly wish I could write here that after that experience I figured things out, and life was great.

But to be honest, it wasn't.

Around me, people thought I was fine and had everything going for me.

I came home after another year of travelling, with my beautiful angel Aroha.

I ended up starting my own little personal training thing in my garage, and made enough money to get by, climbed a bunch of other mountains all over the world and even went to the Himalayas and climbed there.

I came back from Nepal and then went all-in and started my own proper physical gym.

It is even kind of successful...

I even was fortunate to have my parents help support me so we could buy a house.

From the outside looking in, I had everything.

E-V-E-R-Y-T-H-I-N-G

The six pack, the pecs, the awesome girlfriend, the wonderful parents, the car, the house, the fulfilling job, the awesome team, the clients who loved me.

Then, one of the scariest moments of my life happened.

One Tuesday night in Feb 2017.

I was at home on my own, sitting on my bean bag, wearing my dressing gown.

And that feeling.

THAT feeling of hollowness.

Of being alone.

-empty-

That I was absolutely nothing...

That feeling of emptiness, being nothing but that old, rusted bucket...

It all came back again. That same feeling that I had on the beach.

And that after the past ten years of chasing experiences, trying to Do more, Get more, BE more...

With everything I had and experienced...

I was still nothing.

Yes, I ditched the drugs in '07.

I no longer used them to hide.

But since then I had spent the past 10 years trying to BE more.

Chasing a target...

Trying to BE the guy that climbs mountains, the big-balls adventurer.

Trying to BE the traveler, the guy who is self-sufficient and can handle things on his own.

Trying to BE the stud Personal Trainer, the guy who inspires everyone else around him.

Trying to BE the Business Owner, who can manage and run a business, be successful, lead a team and keep his stuff in order.

I was TRYING to be something, a someone. Someone that I thought would eventually leave me feeling Full once I got to the top of this mountain of life I was wanting to climb.

Others around me would look at me and idolised me. I felt like I had more business owners on my email database than clients at one stage, all trying to learn from what I was doing. From the outside looking in everyone was thinking I was crushing it – the beautiful girlfriend, business everyone loved, the pretty car, the nice house, good health.

Many would even tell me things like "man you must be so happy and proud of everything you have created".

That only made things worse. Much worse.

They didn't see the other side.

The training… only as a physical outlet for me to hurt myself, to feel and cause pain – no different than a teenage girl cutting their arm.

The business… that I worked on literally 12-16 hours a day, and on weekends – unable to just relax and chill out and have a break, as that would mean me being alone with my thoughts.

The scarcity… the internal emptiness and the constant pursuit to create, acquire, be more and do more.

The addictions… that began to be my latest self-created outlet from the world that allowed me to be free from all of my thoughts and go into another world.

…The one-dimensional emotionless man that I had self-created.

This is ME.

These were my facts.

This was who I was in my darkness.

So, why do I tell you all this?

You may not be in the same situation, or have the same history, or have the same addictions that I had.

But the challenge is the same.

WE are all the same.

We project forward thinking and feeling and telling ourselves that once we arrive THERE we will be happy.

We don't spend any time getting clear on how we REALLY feel right NOW.

And any of those dark thoughts, or dark places we find ourselves—we never talk about.

We hide them.

From others, but also ourselves.

We suppress them.

And from the suppressing leads us to run a bunch of thoughts and movies in our head about ourselves that aren't true.

They don't serve us. They don't exist.

…They are only created by ourselves!

This book is the script for helping you identify what holds you back, and to help you to finally Stop Stopping.

That old way of starting something new, with good intentions, and smashing it out of the park for a week or two at most if you're lucky… Only to hit a roadblock and be left frustrated, feeling like a failure and eventually giving up. This MUST become a thing of the past.

This book will guide you to embrace what you have already been through, endured, and most importantly, to give you access to the framework that has helped hundreds of our clients break free of what's holding them back so they can get what they want and live a larger life.

People wonder where our motto 'More Than Fitness' comes from. It isn't a sexy tag line that was created over a few espresso shots. Fitness allows the gateway for some experiences into our Selves that many other avenues cannot. But unless we get clear on the other aspects, we are fighting an uphill battle, and all the burpees and broccoli in the world will only allow us to reach 10% of what we are capable of.

Let's begin.

Your first task before we move on is to stare at yourself in a mirror for 60 seconds.

Please don't be 'that guy' who doesn't do anything recommended in a book! I would read books all the time. Feel so accomplished after I got to the end... Only to realise years later that I didn't IMPLEMENT or do the work in hardly any of them! Please learn from my mistakes...

Look in mirror, what do you see and feel?

Why do you think it felt so challenging to just do that?

---

2 THE PAIN FROM THE PAST

*"People are afraid of themselves, of their own reality; their feelings most of all.
People talk about how great love is, but that's bullshit. Love hurts. Feelings are
disturbing. People are taught that pain is evil and dangerous. How can they deal
with love if they're afraid to feel? Pain is meant to wake us up. People try to hide
their pain. But they're wrong. Pain is something to carry, like a radio. You feel
your strength in the experience of pain. It's all in how you carry it. That's what
matters. Pain is a feeling. Your feelings are a part of you. Your own reality. If
you feel ashamed of them, and hide them, you're letting society destroy your reality.
You should stand up for your right to feel your pain."*
— Jim Morrison

"What hurts you, blesses you. Darkness is your candle."
— Jalaluddin Rumi

The human brain does not remember everything, even though we think
it does. We believe the human brain to be a limitless hard drive, that stores
everything that we choose it to from all of our experiences.

But it doesn't.

Yes, you may be able to recall the amazing (and unfortunately the
traumatic) events in your life. You may feel that you are able to recollect
them as if you remember everything about those events. But, the fact is, the
brain only remembers small pieces. It remembers roughly what your friend
said to you, but it does not remember the colour of their tie. You remember
what the meal was, but you forget the contrast of your over-done steak
relative to your 'ok' shiraz that wasn't paired well for the meal.

The same thing happens when we look forward to the future…

Stop for a moment and recognise what happens here. **Anything you think of in the past or future, your brain produces a MOVIE about it in your consciousness.**

Some people call it 'talking to themselves' others call it 'seeing things'. It may not be as vivid as Batman on DVD, but at the end of the day… We create a MOVIE in our minds about what happened in the past or what will happen in the future.

If I tell you I will take you to dinner on the weekend for spaghetti bolognese, you will most likely automatically think of a small, exquisite, Italian restaurant. Your mind will straight away create the setting, the decor, and maybe go as far to imagine an Italian waiter with an accent.

…Oh, how it will all be perfect!

You don't expect the rude waiter, for me to be late, to have to wait 15 minutes for a table, the delay with your entree', the loud obnoxious couple sitting behind you, for your bolognese to be flavorless, to be watery, and for you to get to the end of the night looking at the bill with disgust after feeling like you overpaid way too much for the meal, etc.

This process of self-selecting the good or bad is the same for all the events we have already experienced.

You remember back to your holiday and the good times you had. You forget the boredom you felt after the second week. How the kids behaved half the time. The lack of intimacy you had with your partner, how you began to spend half the day on your phone or doing work…

Likewise, with painful events. You choose to remember all the horrible things that happened, you don't see how it was the catalyst for where you are now, all the good that came from it, who stepped up and supported you instantaneously once you felt the most alone…

So, this is where we will begin. Getting clear on the past. Because unless we can get clear on our past, we can never have a chance of possibly getting clear on what we want for our future.

For YOU…

What are your events?

What in your life now are you still clinging on to?

The supposedly 'good' things that are no longer here?

The 'bad' things that you believe you did that you keep remembering?

What are those events in your life that you constantly think back to?

Feeling anger, pain, guilt, blame, shame, frustration, grief….

Those fleeting thoughts, that always seem to come up…

Those feelings that up until now you have always tried your best to ignore and sedate? Through the food, alcohol and other addictions…

…But they just never seem to go away…

Have some come up? If not take a moment and stop and think a bit deeper.

Here's the crazy thing.

While you believe you may not know where they come from, or maybe you do but you just can't understand why they always seem to pop up at random times…

The truth is they ALWAYS come up at the same time… The same time when everything around you is compounding and getting a too much to handle.

You do your best to ignore it…

But then eventually it all becomes too much… and you explode.

a) on other people – getting angry at your partner, kids, colleagues, friends… for something so small…

b) on yourself – making all those decisions that don't serve you. The mindless tv, the computer games, the beer, the wine, the chocolate, the food, the drugs, the adultery, the sedation…

How has you bottling everything up in your life until now cost you?

Who have you hidden from and said everything is 'ok' or 'good' only to eventually explode? Who felt that? Who were those closest to you that you loved the most that were impacted from you pretending everything is ok? Kids? loved ones? Work colleagues? Family? Friends? You? Your body?

Do you want to be free?

The secret with you being 'happy' is not to lose 10kg, the fix isn't a gym membership... it's working on the 'stuff' that nobody wants to talk about.

You can have Arnold Schwarzenegger train you, have someone prepare and cook you the healthiest meals – and you still won't have success. Not until you recognise and realise what goes through your head, how you deal with those thoughts and most importantly the things you do to sedate yourself when trying to block those thoughts out.

Until you break free of this (this book will help), you will always be living in a vicious cycle. Starting a training program, trying to follow some silly 'diet' and feeling like you are living life sitting on your hands abstaining... You will do good for a week or two, only for these thoughts, feelings and stresses of 'life' to become too much to handle. The end result will be what 90% of the population does and end up with you not training for ages, or going into your cave where you don't want to eat healthy anymore, over eat, eat food that doesn't serve you, drink too much, and give up.

How many times have you gone through this cycle already in your life? If you are like the bulk of our clients who eventually come to us, the answer is too many to count...

Do you want to be free?

Then do the work on the pages in this book.

It's not easy, it's simple.

Not easy. Simple.

Do the work. Don't make this another book where you read the whole book and then curl the ears of pages telling yourself a story saying you will go back – you won't.

Don't make this another book where you speed read so you can get the gratification that it's 'finished'. Finishing doesn't give you growth, only learning does and doing the work.

When the questions come up, please answer them. When you can't find the answers straight away – You stop. You think, you pause, you stop, you think, you pause, and you don't move on until you have the answer.

If the answer is half-assed, you stop, you think, you dig deeper, you answer it more.

-You cannot see what you are capable of until you start to see who you are right now-

So, let's begin.

While we all have MANY things we hold on to from the past, for now we will work on the Main One.

Think about when the shit hits the fan… the overriding story and movie that plays over and over in your mind.

For example;
You just got home, the kids are playing up, you open the mail and the council rates have just arrived and there is already an overdue notice from the water bill. Your friend is being horrible to you at the moment, and your boss had a go at you at work in the morning. Everything feels too much… you just want to break down.

Then the movie begins to play…

While all the above just happened, you cannot help but hear and feel something else about yourself, as part of that movie that is always created by yourself when things get too much… what is it?

For some, it could be as direct as an overriding thought of "I'm a F&$% up!", for others it could be "I'm a terrible mother", "I'm going to lose everything", "I don't deserve what I have", "nobody loves me", "I will always be a failure", etc.

They aren't the nicest things to read, say, hear, or think. But they come up within ourselves all the time. We create these movies inside us on our own. Yet most of the time we choose to not recognise them and do our best to block them out and suppress them (hello food and wine!).

What event in the past are you holding on to, what are the <u>specifics</u> of the event – free of any thoughts or feelings about it? (Be short, concise and to the point)

e.g. - my brother died in 2007. I ran away from home when I was 12. I told my cousin I hated her and she died 2 months later. I was taking drugs for 7 years. I cheated on my partner and had an affair. (*We will use the last one for the follow up questions*).

What feelings and actions come out, when you think of that specific event?

e.g. - I feel angry, annoyed, frustrated, let down, sad, pissed off. I want to run away, cry, quit my life here and never talk to anyone in my family again. (*Due to this being a public book, I kind of need to be nice here, but it's important that you LET OUT whatever is inside you, don't hold back. Let all your dark thoughts and feelings out here*).

When you think about the past event, and clearly see the feelings and actions associated with it… What is the movie that is created in your mind, that YOU are directing, about what happened?

e.g. - I cheated on my partner and had an affair. - then becomes something like; 'I am a horrible person who doesn't deserve to be with my partner. OR it can be the complete opposite 'I cannot find a partner who loves me for who I am'. Don't use my examples or structures. Whatever comes to your mind is RIGHT, it does not matter how good or bad it sounds, just write it down.

What is the <u>COMPLETE OPPOSITE</u> version of that movie above?

e.g. - the original movie: 'I am a horrible person who doesn't deserve to be with my partner. the opposite movie: 'I am a wonderful person who DOES deserve to be with their partner.

_____

_____

_____

What FACTS and TRUTHS are in your life that prove the movie above to be correct? Yes, this is tough when you have feelings of guilt, grief, anger, etc. associated with the original event. But you MUST let go of those feelings for the moment and see the beauty and the gift that is in your life right now for you to move forward. **Really work hard here**. Don't just write one thing. Fill all the lines below, and don't lie to yourself saying you can't find anything. Look harder, deeper.

e.g. - 'I am a wonderful person who DOES deserve to be with their partner. facts & truths: 'I am working through my issues so I can be the best partner I can be. I messed up in the past but love my partner more than ever now. What I did made me realise how much I care about my family. I work so hard and go without so much to provide for them and give them what they want. I am working through this book so I can improve myself.'

_____

_____

_____

_____

_____

_____

_____

If you have done this exercise correct, you will now begin to see a glimmer of hope. That there is a possibility. That maybe there is a space for some brightness in your life, in that same area you used to believe is dark.

Now dream with me, for a moment.

Who would you BE, without the OLD movie, and with complete ownership of the NEW movie? Yes, a tough one again! But put your pen to the paper and see what begins to flow.

e.g. - I would be free to grow, to love those around me, to be my best version of myself, to see the beauty in my wife and kids, to love myself unconditionally and in turn to love them with all their faults also. I would be happy, I would be free of hate.

_____

_____

_____

_____

_____

_____

_____

_____

_____

_____

There are many more movies than just this one.

You MUST continue to be consistent with working through this process for each movie that doesn't serve you.

3 THE DREAM

"The snake which cannot cast its skin has to die. As well the minds which are prevented from changing their opinions; they cease to be mind."
— Friedrich Nietzsche

For 90% of people, the exercise in the previous chapter is HUGE for uncovering the truths about their past. But, once that work is done, a whole new series of movies, beliefs, thoughts, and challenges come up when they think about the future. A whole series of things that don't SERVE us!

And here's the thing, when we are STUCK...

We live in a place either constantly looking back at the PAST, with either guilt or grief;

Guilt - there were more negatives than positives from your actions (e.g. those words I said and the things I did hurt them so much, I can never forgive myself for what I did).

Grief - there were more positives than negatives from the other persons actions (e.g. my loving partner is gone, nobody will love me like they did, I cannot handle life without them)

.... which becomes things like;

GUILT: "I deserve all the suffering I get now, and how I look and feel because of what I DID back then!"
GRIEF: "I would definitely be able to do THAT, if only things were like they used to be in the past!"

Or we live in a place looking forward to the FUTURE with fear or fantasy;

Fear - there will be more negatives than positives from your actions (e.g. If I leave I will lose everything).

Fantasy - there will be more positives than negatives from your actions (e.g. Once I leave my job everything will be perfect)

…. which becomes things like;

FANTASY: "When I lose 10kg I will be happy"

FANTASY: "When work settles down then I can start training and I will be happy"

FANTASY: "I will definitely be able to do THAT, but I just need to wait for THIS to happen first and it will be easy!"

FEAR: "If I lose weight and look sexy, then my partner will get jealous"

FEAR: "If I do that, then people will laugh at me and I will lose my friends"

Where do you live most of your life? (Circle one)

GUILT - GRIEF - FEAR - FANTASY

What is your CURRENT biggest movie about the future? Is it a FEAR or FANTASY?
e.g. - FANTASY: If I get to 70kg I will be happy. FEAR: If I lose weight and start looking pretty my husband will get angry and jealous.

_____

_____

_____

_____

What is the OPPOSITE version of the movie?

e.g. – 'If I get to 70kg I will be happy' - BECOMES – 'If I get to 70kg I won't be happy' (*yes, this is correct and not a typo. If your original thought is that you will be happy, we are balancing your perceptions here by making you contemplate the opposite*). OR…. 'If I lose weight and start looking pretty guys will look at me more and my husband will get angry and jealous' - BECOMES – 'If I lose weight and start looking pretty my husband won't get angry and jealous'.

What FACTS and TRUTHS can prove the OPPOSITE version of the movie to be correct? This isn't about being negative or to make you crazy, it is to help you get polarity and clarity on your thoughts and balance your perceptions so you can move forward.

e.g. – 'If I get to 70kg I won't be happy' = 'I won't be happy simply by looking a certain way, I will be happy by changing how I feel about myself as a whole. By becoming a confident person who accepts myself for who I am, and uncovering beliefs that hold me back, like in this book.' OR 'If I lose weight and start looking pretty my husband won't get angry and jealous' = 'My husband won't feel that way if I share my real reasons for why I am doing it, that I am doing it for him and the kids to set an example, and so I personally feel more confident so I can be myself more and also so I can feel sexier in bed and when I am around him.'

Hopefully now you can see the complete CHAOS that comes from having beliefs from the PAST that hold you back as a VICTIM in some way, shape or form. As well as beliefs in the FUTURE that aren't completely true either.

How many opportunities have you lost? How much hard work has been undone? How many times have you chosen to be placed in your own PRISON? The prison YOU created? The prison that never existed except within your own mind? How much has it cost you? Who would you be, if you were free from it? How old are you, how many years have you been living with feelings of guilt and grief in your life? And how many years have you been living with fear and fantasy in your future? What pain do you feel? Don't hold back! Go to town and write it all out!

_____

_____

_____

_____

_____

_____

_____

_____

_____

_____

_____

_____

_____

Why must you decide to move forward NOW? Why must you do this for YOU? What must you CHOOSE to do? How do you feel about the possibility of the POWER that can come from you CHOOSING to finally COMMIT to this?

_____

_____

_____

_____

_____

_____

_____

_____

REMEMBER: **From PAIN comes POWER**.

4 THE PRESENT

"Yesterday is gone. Tomorrow has not yet come. We have only today. Let us begin."
— Mother Teresa

You have now began to recognise some of the cataclysmic events from the past.

That caused pain.

Suffering.

That didn't SERVE you.

You have seen your false beliefs about the future.

That made you see unclear.

That caused hesitation.

Resistance.

But now...

Now you have more clarity.

More clarity with your past and future. And the thoughts that are associated.

So, let's talk about NOW.

Right now – This moment.

The PRESENT.

Where you are, right now, reading this book in your hands?

What are the FACTS AND TRUTHS about this moment, with your body?

e.g. - I am 30kg overweight. Take depression medication 2x/day. Take fluid tablets. I get tired every day at 3pm. I don't feel confident wearing a suit or at the beach. I don't feel attractive to my partner. I use coffee to keep me awake. I drink 8 beers a night. I don't play with my kids because I have no energy. I get stressed easily.

_____

_____

_____

_____

What has been the COST associated to you being like this? How has it impacted opportunities in your life, events and the people around you that you care about?

e.g. - I have missed opportunities at work due to holding myself back because I don't want to speak in front of people. I have missed making memories with my son in his youngest years. I have drifted away from my partner. I have let my parents down. I have made others in my family learn my bad habits. I have wasted thousands of dollars on medication.

_____

_____

_____

_____

How does that make you FEEL?

_____

_____

_____

_____

Hopefully you have been answering the questions and going all-in until now (if you haven't, STOP and go back! Otherwise you are wasting your time).

But now it's time to shift gears and begin to talk about all the things that seem to just pop up and upset us on a daily basis. The events that flood us with those emotions that make us contract in anger and frustration with those around us. And, most importantly, to share the process that allows you to break free from this happening once and for all.

So, when was the last time you made a conscious choice of your own free will, to HURT someone you really cared about?

That conscious choice to make your loved one angry and upset, when you knew they did nothing to deserve it—simply because you just felt like it?

You might be like most people and say the words…

NEVER!!! I WOULD N-E-V-E-R DO THAT!!!

WHO DO YOU THINK I AM!!!!

…it's interesting, isn't it? We would NEVER do something like that, but for some strange reason… everyone else that we know in this world seems to do it to us!

I am going to go a little left field now. But stay with me.

Right now, there are atrocities happening overseas with groups like ISIS doing things to people that are unimaginable. Choosing to select a person who has done nothing to them, torture them and do unthinkable acts of brutality like decapitating their head all while recording it for the rest of the world to see...

It is easy to point the finger and say how despicable they are. "Animals! What is wrong with these people!".

And I am not here to argue with that for one moment, or where the world seems to be headed...

BUT...

WHY do they do it?

When we remove the first layer and say they are animals. The second layer of passing blame to their religion, the third layer of blaming their nationality, and start to get to a deeper cause...

We begin to POSSIBLY get to their pain.

The pain from them being VICTIMS to other people in their life.

The bombs dropped on their towns years and years ago from previous wars. When they would look around and see deformed people from bomb blasts. The sister who walked to the shops but never came back. A life they lived that is completely incomprehensible to most of the western world.

And the movie THEY told THEMSELVES why it happened. "All they want is our oil!" "they do not want what is best for us, they just want our country!".

The pain builds up.

People share the pain.

A tribe forms.

A leader speaks.

A movement begins.

And a (stupid) idea to try and fix the pain and relieve the suffering is birthed.

An idea where they believe deep in their core that by doing this now, eventually the pain will stop. That the other countries will leave them alone, the wars will stop, the bombs will stop, and they will be left to their own devices.

Hopefully the above horrific situation can help us see that even in those extreme circumstances they would not necessarily occur if there wasn't a catalyst that starts it all.

So, if we can have awareness that maybe our beliefs of other people, things and events, small things, minor things, like;

-when your work colleague looks at you funny
-when your partner yells at you for leaving your socks out on the kitchen floor
-when your client gives you a bad review
-when your child never makes her bed
-when your wife keeps nagging you
-when your husband doesn't thank you
-when your sister never messages you for your birthday
-when your boss never thanks you for completing your work on time

Maybe, just maybe….

It isn't done on purpose and them coming from that place to just make you feel terrible and upset. That they aren't selfish, arrogant, weird, hateful…

Consider the possibility, that every single time something small like the above happens to you. That it is NEVER done on purpose to upset you, that it is not their FAULT. That YOU have created the feelings inside of yourself based on areas of YOUR life that you are yet to LEARN and GROW from. That in some weird and wonderful way you have created all this chaos inside your mind and given yourself these feelings as a conscious choice. From a movie you have ran in YOUR mind. A movie you have created without realising.

Time for me to share a recent experience (I'm not a psychopath – I promise!)

The day I thought my coach shat on me

5:45am Tuesday Morning

It was a cold winters morning, the gym was super busy, considering how cold it was (I am always so blown away with our clients' commitment, in a world where most people think we are getting lazier and lazier…)

I was doing Personal Training with one of our longest serving clients.

One of my other amazing coaches (Let's call them PT2) was doing Personal Training with a newer client. She had only been with us around 6 weeks.

Another two coaches were running the group training.

We had been all coaching since 5:30am…

And then, at 5:45am, PT2 went to the toilet.

I saw this happen out of the corner of my eye.

While his client was left there on the floor doing some mobility drills.

FACT: PT2 just went to the toilet while he had a client to train.

What feelings came to me straight away?

FEELINGS: Anger, frustration, annoyance.

What was the movie that I created in my mind that I told myself about the event? After the facts happened and the feelings came over me?

MOVIE: PT2 doesn't care about our clients and doesn't care about doing a good job here.

What actions do I want to do after I told myself that movie?

ACTIONS: I want to run over to the toilet, bang on the door and smash it in! I want to shout at them! I want to yell and ask them "what the hell do you think you are doing? You have a client paying a premium amount for a premium service and they don't deserve to have a coach like you do a shit while they are meant to be trained!" I

want to punch them in the face! (*I am not crazy I promise*)

Except I don't do that right then in that moment.

I keep it internalised.

Drive myself a little crazy.

And in the past, I wouldn't say anything. Just suppress it all... Be weird around them for the next few days.

That was then.

Now something different happens...

But before we go there – can you see this process happening in your daily life?

Fact: child doesn't make bed.
Feel: angry, upset.
Movie: that your child never listens to you.
Actions: you want to get angry at them, and maybe that you also want to give up even trying as a parent.

Fact: friend left party without saying bye.
Feel: sad, lonely, neglected.
Movie: that your friend doesn't like you.
Actions: you never want to talk to them again.

Fact: partner works late and doesn't spend time with the kids.
Feel: sad, annoyed, frustrated, angry, upset.
Movie: that your partner doesn't love you or care about the kids.
Actions: you want to leave them and find someone who supports and appreciates you more.

Now, let's go back to my coach (PT2) and his little toilet break.

The Fact still happens.

The Feeling still happens.

The Movie still happens.

(All within a few seconds)

But now, as soon as the movie happens, the movie that is automatically created by those facts and feelings…

I ask myself a new question.

What is the opposite movie?

Then all of a sudden, something strange happens.

"PT2 doesn't care about our clients and doesn't care about doing a good job here" becomes;

OPPOSITE MOVIE: PT2 does care about our clients and does care about doing a good job here

And, while I am having the chaotic recipe of feelings flowing through my blood of anger, frustration and annoyance… It is hard to believe it.

But I don't want to be right. I want to get what I want.

And what I want is to balance my emotions, and to be in control. (And to not be that crazy psychopath that you probably think I already am)

So, I ask myself another question. After I have the opposite version.

What FACTS and TRUTHS do I have to PROVE that opposite movie true?

"Where recently has PT2 unquestionably shown that they do care about our clients and that they do care about doing a good job here?"

Then all of a sudden, like a shower of love, clarity, beauty and peace raining down on me…

Something divine happens.

I begin to SEE. I begin to see the beauty of that person.

In that moment, after the feelings of anger, frustration and annoyance washed over me…

They begin to dissipate, as I begin to see what they just recently did.

Where only last week they worked for 14 hours every day for 5 days in a row, making a choice to miss out on their training because they were so engrossed in the latest project they were given and the amazing job they wanted to do and to completely over-deliver by the deadline date.

Where they came in on the previous Saturday to have a consult with one of their clients and check in because they hadn't seen them in a couple of weeks due to personal issues.

Where they independently started to research and sign up for a new course to improve their knowledge on nutrition.

All of a sudden.

No more anger, frustration, annoyance.

Just the ability afterwards to ask a question and see what was going on.

In this case, the poor coach had a gastro bug and didn't want to let the team or client down first thing in the morning and have a sickie.

He went above ALL expectations and came in, while sick... So the client was looked after.

All of a sudden, even after running through this process, asking myself these questions to arrive at a place where I was more balanced in my emotions, thoughts and beliefs about them...

Then came the recognition and realisation that the <u>ORIGINAL event in itself</u> was the perfect example of the highest level of commitment. Higher than even the opposite version of the movie that I went through this processes with.

That nothing upsetting was done at all by the coach – except for what I created personally in my own mind.

That ALL of my suffering and feelings of contraction were created by MYSELF out of something that NEVER existed.

And the crazy thing... This is just one small example, that came from a coach going to the toilet.

This happens ALL the time.

EVERY day.

These THOUGHTS, FEELINGS and ACTIONS that come from MOVIES that DON'T serve you – Happen all the time!

The small things like your partner not listening to you, to the big things like you getting yelled at in front of all your work colleagues.

But the process is the same.

I want you to consider the possibility, of how life would be, if you owned this process, and you had a way to arrive at place each time free of those emotions that make you contract...

And you can just see the real underlying truth in the events.

Who would you be?

How would you feel?

What would you NOT need to do?

Would you NEED to visit that dark place?

The place that is the home to all the things that DON'T serve you in your life?

The excess food.
The food you eat that you know makes you unhealthy.
The soft drink.
The wine.
The beer.
The mindless TV.
The computer games.
The excessive spending on material things that make you happy for only a moment.
That place you go where you don't talk and share your feelings at all.
That place where you blow up and explode on those around you for the tiniest of things.

Who would you be without all that?

It might sound overwhelming.

Like it is incomprehensible to think that is a possibility.

But it isn't.

All it takes is a commitment. A commitment to ask yourself some simple questions, when you feel yourself contracting.

Do this right now.

Look back to the last event that upset you (I am sure you don't have to think far back!).

What are the specific facts of that event?

_____

_____

_____

_____

How did you feel?

_____

_____

_____

What is the movie you are playing to yourself?

_____

_____

_____

_____

What is the OPPOSITE version of that movie?

_____

_____

_____

_____

What FACTS and TRUTHS do you have that prove the OPPOSITE version to be true?

_____

_____

_____

_____

_____

_____

You must go through this process every time something triggers you!

This may take some time at the beginning, but it will get easier as you continue to be consistent with the process. It is definitely not as hard as walking around with all of those chaotic thoughts in your mind every day that don't serve you!

Make sure you access the free resources and bonuses for this book at 365performance.com.au/book. You are able to download these questions as a printout so you can do the work at any time.

If you don't be consistent with this process and tell yourself you will be 'ok'... These small minor events that upset you will continue to happen like they always have in the past.

And over time they will begin to stack up on top of each other like they always have...

That person not listening to you, you not having enough time, you not feeling supported, you feeling stressed. And that movie that doesn't serve you keeps playing…

Then this strange thing happens.

Which is those 'minor' movies related to those person(s) or event(s).

Begins to morph and transform.

Into the darker version.

It's the one that goes through your head as you dive into that dark place where you sedate yourself with all those things that don't serve you, that we discussed at the beginning of the book.

That same movie that makes you contract into your cocoon.

Those horrible things you tell yourself like "I'm a F&$% up!", "I'm a terrible mother", "I'm going to lose everything", "I don't deserve what I have", "nobody loves me", "I will always be a failure", etc.

The movie that has played all your life.

From your PAST.

That 'craving' for alcohol, sweets, tv, porn, computer games, eating rubbish becomes unbearable…

And you end up back in that dark place you find yourself in, so you don't 'feel'.

And you give in and give up.

Arriving back at the mercy of the same movie that has never served you.

Do you see now how all your life you have been running the same loop with everything you ever wanted? Up until now always being held ransom to 'life' from the same old movie?

You have been held back by an anchor you have created in your own mind.

It was never anyone else around you.

Never your boss, your kids, your partner, your friend, your colleague…

That no matter who they were, even if they left and were no longer there…

You always found someone else who would make you feel that 'charge'…

One person would leave but another would show up.

The same feelings…

That would transform into the story from your past.

But not anymore.

Ask the questions and be FREE.

In summary, when you don't feel good about something;

What are the facts?
What am I feeling?
What is the movie I am playing to myself?
What is the opposite version of that movie?
What facts and truths do I have that prove this to be true?

You do not need a new meal plan.
You do not need to train 7 days a week.
You are not different.
You are not destined to be 'that' way.
You are not a victim.
You just need to get clear in your mind.

You are worthy.

You have permission.

5 THE UNWRAPPING

"We can easily forgive a child who is afraid of the dark;
the real tragedy of life is when men are afraid of the light."
— Plato

This book is in your hand.

It has been painful to read.

It has been painful to think.

It has been painful to do the work.

And above all, it has been most painful—to really feel...

But you're here.

And if you have done the work.

You will right now have a fire burning deep inside.

Not a fire of victim or circumstance.

But a fire of purpose and desire.

That you created...

Here's the thing. As humans, it is much easier to move AWAY from pain, than to move TOWARDS pleasure.

Religion is so successful because they get people in because they DON'T want to go to hell. Once they are indoctrinated then they begin to move towards wanting to go to heaven (or wherever else you want to be going).

…It is also why around 80% of people who try to start an exercise program to 'look good' don't have the most success. Because they are focusing on moving TO pleasure – not AWAY from pain.

Hopefully this is beginning to make sense now, it is why I have spent over 8,000 words in this book to hopefully make you understand your own pain a little more.

We have (hopefully) done that now.

And while we are almost there, there are still a couple of things that still hold us back, a few hangers-on, that if not addressed, will cloud what you want.

Because from your past experiences, stories, events…

And the (sometimes) lack of results.

You have created labels for yourself somewhat unknowingly.

LAZY.

UNMOTIVATED.

Things like the above that don't serve you.

That aren't true…

'Laziness' and 'not motivated' aren't traits that you are born with. They come from a lack of results from the work put in.

"I am lazy and not motivated to save money"—when I feel like I am living on SPAM and rice for 4 weeks and then have no savings to show for it at the end of the month.

"I am lazy and not motivated to lose weight"—when I diet like crazy, am hungry all the time, train hard and don't see any results or cannot sustain it.

I want you to consider the possibility using the example above, that if all you did was train 3x/week – maybe at a gym or simply go for a walk. And you ate relatively well – food that tasted nice, wasn't bland, and you never felt hungry, nor were you buying food that was any more expensive...

And you made consistent progress to your goals week after week...

(This happens every single week with our clients by the way)

Would you be lazy and unmotivated anymore?

No.

Why?

Because there was an OUTCOME from your EFFORT. You weren't doing too much too soon and the effort wasn't unmanageable. You were able to consistently see your body transform, which allows you to have more belief in yourself from knowing that from the tiny lifestyle changes you do make, they are getting you what you want.

So, get clear. And answer the below questions.

Starting with the first one.

Which is SIMPLE.

But not EASY.

What do you want?

Let it flow.

Think about what you want;

With your body & health
With your family & children
With your work & finances
With your relationships
With yourself & god

Fill the next page.

What do you want?

Why do you want it?

_____

_____

_____

_____

_____

_____

_____

_____

_____

_____

_____

_____

_____

_____

_____

_____

_____

_____

Now for the thing that is never discussed.

Resistance.

You get busy with work, the kids are sick, there are too many bills to pay, your partner isn't supporting you, your friends are telling you to stop being so much of a health nut, the traffic is bad, you're tired, you need to travel for work…

And all you feel you can do is stop, not train, not work on your nutrition or your health.

…And all you would do in the past is exactly that… STOP… and give in to the resistance.

The resistance – which is just 'life'.

You will always be busy, and 'life' will always get in the way.

But the reason why life gets in the way for everyone, but some people still manage to have success with their health, relationships, finances, etc…

Is because they have a big WHY.

So….

When 'life' happens, and things get in the way, it starts to get too much, and you feel like you can't make it through the resistance, why must you push through?

_____

_____

_____

_____

_____

_____

What would life look like in 5 years if you don't begin to make a change now?

_____

_____

_____

_____

_____

What would life look like in 10 years if you don't begin to make a change now?

_____

_____

_____

_____

_____

What would life look like in 20 years if you don't begin to make a change now?

_____

_____

_____

_____

_____

There is no secret to anything.

If you look back through history.

At any of the greats.

The smartest did not finish university.

The passionate did not grow up smothered in love.

The healthiest did not grow up with it being their life.

The wealthiest did not grow up with it being inherited.

The most spiritual did not grow up with a relationship with god.

They created it.

From a big why.

An unrelenting commitment to what they wanted to accomplish.

Fueled by a recognition of their past.

And an internal desire to BE the change, not WAIT for it.

Me.

You.

We.

Can all learn from them.

It all starts with one thing.

Giving ourselves the PERMISSION to begin to make it happen.

You deserve to get what you want.

You have a choice now – to not wait for a bad report from the Doctor or a horrible event to happen to you to force you to change – but for you to initiate it now, from your own free will.

Why must you finally give yourself the permission to execute on the life you want?

_____

_____

_____

_____

_____

_____

_____

_____

_____

_____

_____

_____

_____

_____

_____

_____

6 THE PURPOSE

"Man often becomes what he believes himself to be. If I keep on saying to myself that I cannot do a certain thing, it is possible that I may end by really becoming incapable of doing it. On the contrary, if I have the belief that I can do it, I shall surely acquire the capacity to do it even if I may not have it at the beginning."
— Mahatma Gandhi

After completing the work up until now and recognising things from the past and the old way you used to view the future, you should now have a feeling inside you of what you want to create, who you want to be, and most importantly a deep fire and a KNOWING that you can make it happen.

Now it's time to get clearer on that.

Time to see it, feel it, taste it.

Most likely for the first time in your life.

Close your eyes and imagine.

When you accomplish all that you are after.

How do you look...?
How do you feel...?
How do you carry yourself in social situations...?

Get clearer.

After finally having ARRIVED...

What is that MOMENT?

Where are you? Outside? Inside?

What is the event? Your family Christmas? Work presentation? Catching up with friends you haven't seen in a while?

What's the weather like? Hot? Cold? Warm? Raining? Overcast?

What are you wearing? A dress? Singlet? Skirt? Jacket?

Who's there? Family? Friends? People you haven't seen before?

What's it smell like?

What are you doing?

How are people looking at you?

How are you feeling when you walk in there? Proud? Energised? Enthusiastic? Confident? In control? Powerful?

What do people say to you? Do they say it as a group? Or come up individually?

How do their comments make you feel?

How does the way they look at you, make you feel?

How do you react?

Close your eyes and see it in your mind's eye.

Feel it.

Let it be part of you.

Let it soak into your blood.

Take note of everything. And Write!

Where are you? What do you see? Be specific!

_____

_____

_____

_____

_____

_____

_____

Now it's time for us to move forward and see the impact you will have on not only your life, but those around you. Time to understand how when you achieve what you want and continue living it for the rest of your life, how it will impact yourself, your family, and all those you care about.

What will life look like in 5 years if you finally begin to make a change now and live the life you know you must? How will things be different in 5 years for not only you, but those around you? How will your experiences be different? How will the lives of those around you be better? How much more purposeful and fulfilled will you be?

_____

_____

_____

_____

_____

_____

What would life look like in 10 years after creating this life that you believe you must? Imagine yourself staring into your own eyes in a mirror. How would you feel knowing that you succeeded and that after all those years of stopping, you made a choice 10 years ago that shaped you forever? How proud do you feel? What have you experienced? What do other people think of you after understanding all you have accomplished?

_____

_____

_____

_____

_____

What would life look like in 20 years after creating the life you truly desire? You may be a little wrinkly now, maybe there are grandkids. How do you feel knowing you made choices earlier in your life to allow you to be here today and know you still have many years left? Looking back on the past 20 years and all you have accomplished and experienced, how do you feel knowing you lived life to its fullest?

_____

_____

_____

_____

_____

_____

How many lives will you impact from living true to yourself and on purpose? WHO will benefit from you being focused in following your path and getting what you want? HOW will your actions end up serving them? Think of 4 people you care about and list who they are and how your actions will impact them for the better.

Who? _____

How?

_____

_____

Who? _____

How?

_____

_____

Who? _____

How?

_____

_____

Who? _____

How?

_____

_____

7 THE PATH

"If you do not change direction, you may end up where you are heading"
— Gautama Buddha

Having success is simple.

Not easy, simple.

Right now, there is an area of your life that is pretty awesome.

And from it being 'awesome, you would tell me "It's not that hard!".

Maybe it is your relationship? It's simple you say! Just prioritise having quality time with them, being open, and sharing how you feel!

Maybe it is your spirituality? It's simple you say! Make time for it every day, and on the weekend, go to church!

Maybe it is your business? It's simple you say! Do what you are good at, and delegate the rest!

With your health and fitness and nutrition it is no different;

Move a bit more – relative to how much you are moving at the moment.
Eat a bit better – relative to what you are eating at the moment.

It's not hard, but we build our own prison and create our own chaos of complexity...

BUT! BUT! BUT! BUT! How much better? I must eat perfect! And how many grams of protein relative to my bodyweight? What types of carbs? Low GI or High GI? What is the fat content of steak? If I eat too many eggs will I have cholesterol problems? Is bacon bad? How many calories in a banana?

And because we don't have all the answers we don't do anything.

Or, we do begin… and then we make a small mistake and give up.

But it's simple.

Move a bit more – relative to how much you are moving at the moment.

Eat a bit better – relative to what you are eating at the moment.

In the coming pages, we will give you some guidelines on how you can begin to improve your health and see success.

It is not rocket science. And the biggest fallacy of the health and wellness industry is that it needs to be. It doesn't…

We have achieved such amazing results with our clients from making the complex simple. The advice on these pages has, at the time of writing, helped over 2,238 of our clients have success over the years.

Make sure you check out our amazing clients success stories on our website **365performance.com.au**.

It worked for them, and it will help you also – if you allow it.

8 EAT

"Let food be thy medicine and medicine be thy food."
— Hippocrates

"What should I eat?"

If you have any health issues you may find, like so many of our clients, that working on this first part of your health can be completely life changing.

Unlike most who treat the SYMPTOMS with pills, by addressing your health with your nutrition, you begin to treat the underlying CAUSE.

While every person out there who is wanting to create a name for themselves will lead you to believe that what you need is a specific supplement, or a uniquely tailored macronutrient plan for your body, the truth is, for 95% of the population, you want to simply limit the things that don't serve you, and increase the consumption of the things that do.

If you are like most people;
You eat too much processed food and sugar with hardly any nutritional value.
You under eat vegetables, protein and healthy fats—the things that give your body what it needs to perform optimally.

So every day you keep eating these foods that have no nutritional value. Your body doesn't get what it really needs, so craves more food. You keep feeling hungry all the time – not due to the amount of food you put it, but due to the quality of it. From your body not getting what it wants and needs it tells you to put more food in – you think you are hungry and need more 'food' when what is really happening is you are nutrient deprived and simply need to begin to eat better 'quality' food.

The mindset of what we will be discussing here is PROGRESS not PERFECTION.

So many people come to me, never training before, eating nothing but processed foods and soft drink for the past 10 years. They begin to eat healthy, and slip up for one meal on the weekend and think they are a failure.

...they have had more healthy meals in one week then they have in the past 10 years! That is not failure!

NEWSFLASH: I still drink alcohol every now and then (I am a margarita man), I will enjoy a slice of cake when it is someone's birthday, and I may even get desert when I go to a nice dinner with my partner!

Your life is there to be enjoyed! You begin to put on weight and not have success when these 'treats' become daily events.

But before we start...

The first piece we need to identify and recognise is that until now... even if I wrote you up a personalised meal plan, relative to all the lovely foods you like to eat, with healthy options, so you literally just follow it to the letter and see success (which we do with our clients at 365 Performance). And EVEN if you had the funds to have someone cook everything for you, so you never had to worry about cooking and preparing food ever again...

If we gave you all the above, there would still be all the circumstances and events in your life that would still annoy and upset you. Over time, they would stack up like they always do and became too much to handle, leaving you stressed, angry and upset...

Then the viscous cycle would still occur. After following the plan for a week or two, you would normally not be aware of all those feelings, etc. It would all be too much, you will give in with the same OLD MOVIE you always had and go back to your old way.

It is important to identify now before we go any deeper that when this happens, the feelings of chaos and struggle in your life – and it will happen – that you get clear on what the movie is that is playing and you run through and work the process that we have already discussed in the earlier chapters so you can get out of this rut, find the learning, and keep progressing!

Let's begin.

Our first aim is to REPLACE the foods that don't serve us with the things that do.

NOTICE what I just said.

REPLACE.

It sounds foreign to most people who have been told they need to CUT and REMOVE everything.

It automatically puts us on the back-burner because we feel like we are missing out.

SOFT DRINKS & JUICES:
Coke, Solo, Pepsi, Fanta etc... all of these drinks are full of sugar. Your next question will undoubtedly be something along the lines of "but I drink Coke Zero". If it looks like rubbish, smells like rubbish, it means it is. Without getting technical, these other ingredients that create the same taste as sugar but don't have the actual ingredient to make the side of the can look as bad, they still have the same impact on certain chemicals in the brain and body that make you crave certain things. Not to mention we don't know how harmful these things really are to us long term.

"But juice is good for me". While a serving of fruit a day can definitely be beneficial to most people, in most fruit juices the amount of sugar is even higher than in soft drink. Yes, the sugars may come from fruit, but for most people wanting to lose weight, it doesn't matter if the sugar comes from a fruit or not, it is still excess calories that don't serve you in getting to your goal.

COFFEE & TEA:
We have no issues with coffee and tea, just with a lot of the fillers that people put in them!

There is a difference between a long black, or an espresso shot – vs a large mocha frappe. One has 0 calories, the other has 500+!

Likewise with tea, no issues with green tea, black tea – but if you get a tea and put 5 teaspoons of sugar in, that is an issue.

So, what should you drink instead?

Water. You can add lemon or lime to make it taste nicer. Alternatively, if you miss the 'fizz' from the soda you can drink soda water.

It's that simple.

Whenever you feel like a coke – have a soda water. If you feel like a juice, drink some water… Any time you are thirsty, drink soda water or water.

"Is that all?"

Yes. And the crazy thing, relative to some people I know who can drink up to 2L+ of soft drink, cordial, or juice a day…

This simple tweak can lead them to lose 1+kg/week consistently, without changing anything else.

For the coffee drinkers – try to have your coffee black with no milk, if that is tough just try limit the milk. e.g. maybe go from having a large coffee with milk to a small coffee or a piccolo with milk but keep the same amount of shots in it if you like.

Likewise, for the tea drinkers – try having green tea.

HAVE PROTEIN WITH EVERY MEAL:
For most meals, the majority of people eat way too many carbs and way too little protein.

Right now, I want you to imagine there were three of you.

Locked in your own jail cell.

Person one got a bowl with 200g of carbs (say rice, bread, or pasta).

Person two got a bowl with 200g of fats (say almonds, walnuts, or cashews).

Person three got a bowl with 200g of protein (say salmon, steak, or chicken).

Then you were locked away for the next 48 hours. No more food.

If that was the case, Person one would get hungry first (with the carbs). Then person two (with the fats), then person three (with the protein).

...Why?

Because protein has the highest satiety value of all the macronutrients (protein, carbs and fat).

...What does that mean?

Of all the different types of foods, protein keeps you the fullest for longest.

...What does that mean?

If you eat protein at every meal, you will stay fuller for longer, which will lead to you not eating as much food.

...What does that mean?

You will eat less calories than you normally do and you will lose weight.

"So, what protein should I put in my meals?"

If it walks, swims, or flies – eat it!

Some ideas;

Land: Pork, beef, lamb, kangaroo.
Sea: Tuna, salmon, barramundi, crab.
Air: Chicken, turkey, duck.

Right now, you are undoubtedly thinking about having a rib eye steak for breakfast at 5am and feel like telling me to go jump. I get it.

The above are the protein sources in their simplest form, but there are a bunch of variants and easier options, relative to your situation, circumstance and time available.

High quality slices of the above chicken, turkey, etc. are a great choice from the deli.

As is mince, good quality bacon, omega-3 enriched eggs and even things like gourmet sausages are ok…

If you are vegan some options are tofu, tempeh, vegan (pea and rice) protein powders, beans / legumes.

Yes, the idea of grass-fed, organic, free range, etc. are all better choices… but just focus on doing what you can here. And remember the main mindset for this section – PROGRESS not PERFECTION!

You want to think of all the choices you can make as being the equivalent of sitting on a pyramid scale. The top choice is some sort of grass fed organic steak that has been massaged by a monk that only ever ate anything that was pure. But there is also the bottom of the pyramid which is the equivalent of what most people have which is high calorie, nutrient empty foods like white bread, coke and sauce.

Our goal is to begin to get you a little higher up the pyramid.

So don't overthink it. Just add some protein to every meal.

If you are still lost, don't worry – we will make it all come together soon!

VEGETABLES:
For most people in this day and age, 'vegetable' is the swear word of the 21st century. For most meals vegetables and salad are pretty much nonexistent.

And to tell you the truth, this was pretty much the same for me.

I never was a fan of them…

And I never really knew what an impact it was having on my health, as it seemed to just be 'how I felt' all the time.

But that's the thing with our health. We always have a bunch of things that are COMMON but not NORMAL.

It's COMMON to not go to the toilet every day – but not NORMAL.

It's COMMON to go to the toilet and spray the bowl – but not NORMAL.

It's COMMON to walk around bloated, fart all the time, be constipated – but not NORMAL.

The majority of the time it comes from poor gut health.

And one of the largest contributing factors is from the lack of fiber and nutrients in the gut – which vegetables are the largest provider of.

So, your focus is to eat MORE veg.

How much? More than you do at the moment.

For some of you, it may literally be something as small as eating a handful of spinach at every meal.

For some of you, it may be making sure you have half a plate worth of vegetables with every meal.

Just know where you are at, and do a little bit MORE.

For your vegetables, in a perfect world they should be local and organic! But don't drive 4 hours to make this happen or pay $20 for a broccoli stem. Just shop with the season, which typically means what is on sale and mix up the colours for extra points (e.g. don't just eat 2kg of broccoli every day of your life).

PRO TIP: If you are anything like me, and you didn't even know what a vegetable was from your younger years, a great way to get a surge of veg into you in a simple way is to make yourself a smoothie.

Notice I said SMOOTHIE not juice – if you juice the vegetable all the fiber is taken out – which is all of the good stuff.

Get 250-500ml water. Get a bunch of vegetables – I would get a whole bag of spinach (yes, seriously), kale, carrot, celery, ginger, cucumber, add 1/2 a cup of blueberries for taste, and some protein powder, blend it up and drink that.

It made me feel amazing. My guts worked the best they ever had, I began to have the best experience in the toilet – but also my skin began to look amazing and my mental clarity and energy went through the roof!

FRUIT:
Fruit is one of those foods that so many people consume when they are wanting to lose weight, THINKING they are being healthy but a lot of the time are completely destroying their chances of success.

There is nothing wrong with fruit but most of it is extremely high in fructose (sugar).

Which means when people are trying to improve their diet and cutting back on excess carbs they end up consuming them unknowingly from fruit instead.

I see so many people who come to me and are eating clean, but then at lunch they are having a huge fruit salad, snacking on fruit all through the day and wondering why they aren't losing weight.

Once they change this they begin to progress again.

So, if your goal is to lose weight you want to limit fruit to 1 serving/day (PS – one serving is not a whole watermelon!). Preferably consume the fruit after you exercise. Berries like blueberries, strawberries, blackberries etc. are your best bet.

FATS:
If 'vegetables' was a foreign word for some people, 'fats' is another one. And the media doesn't do much to help!

'FAT FREE' – So many people see this and believe it is a better choice. But, when you read the label and see how much SUGAR is in there instead, you begin to realise that isn't the case.

You want to be having HEALTHY fats in your diet.

Healthy fats not only provide your body with energy but also help move the vitamins A, D, E and K through your bloodstream and absorb them into your body. The essential fatty acids also play a role in brain development, blood clotting, reproductive health and managing inflammation, among other things.

Don't be scared of healthy fats.

I am not wanting you to drink dirty chip fat from the local take-away.

I am talking about having things like olive oil in your salad, eating almonds, walnuts, cashews, avocado, coconut milk, etc.

Simply add a small serving to every meal.

ALCOHOL:
"Oh no, he isn't going to bring this up, is he?"

First and foremost, after doing the work at the beginning of the book you should be more aware of the things that make you want to drink.

Recognise there are times when you feel like having a glass, vs having a whole bottle.

When you feel like drinking heaps and writing yourself off there are normally a bunch of feelings and movies running through your mind that you are suppressing.

So, get clear on that first.

But, when you do want to go out and have a drink and make the best choice possible, you want to limit beer and other drinks high in calories, like all those pre-mixed drinks.

Some better choices are;
365 'Skinny' – White spirit (tequila, etc.) with soda water and a heap of FRESH lime

Red wine like Pinot noir, merlot, etc.

Another tip is to drink a glass or two of water between each alcoholic drink. It not only spreads out the time between drinks but also helps keep you hydrated.

SERVING SIZES:
How many meals should you have? How often should you eat?

While many can benefit from having a uniquely tailored plan (which we do for our clients) there are some general guidelines that can get you extremely close to what your body needs without being complicated.

For a great starting point, we use the Precision Nutrition guidelines and use your hands for portion sizing of meals.

Please note the below is not only width but thickness also. Don't overthink it and drive yourself crazy. Nobody became obese from having 2g extra of steak or one extra almond.

Your palm determines your protein portion – One palm for ladies, two palms for males.

Your fist determines your vegetable portion – One fist for ladies, two fists for males.

Your thumb determines your fat portion – One thumb for ladies, two thumbs for males.

And for those who are having them, your cupped hand determines your starchy carbohydrate portion (preferably after training) – One handful for ladies, two handfuls for males.

Once the above is on your plate, ensure you are practicing mindful eating (not just scoffing it down while watching the Simpsons). Don't overthink it! Just chew your food, eat slowly and to 80% full.

Satiety takes around 20 min to kick in, so by eating slowly and chewing your food your body doesn't only absorb the nutrients better but you also reduce your chances of overeating.

The above is the simplest way to have balanced meals. When first doing this, you may not be hungry for 5-8 hours after eating, or you may be hungry after two hours. Simply eat when hungry, and practice the above principles and you will be making progress.

MEAL IDEAS:
It doesn't need to be hard. Just think PROTEIN / VEG / FAT.

Most meals should look something like this:
-A serving of healthy protein such as chicken, lean beef, turkey, pork or salmon
-A serving of mixed vegetables like cucumber, broccoli, tomato, spinach or cauliflower.
-Some healthy fats like olive oil, a small thumb of almonds, or avocado.

Breakfast may be;
-3 eggs and some spinach.
-slices of turkey breast, 1/2 an avocado and broccoli with olive oil.
-a green smoothie with kale, spinach, protein powder, coconut milk.

Lunch/dinner may be;
-chicken salad with olive oil.
-salmon and veg with some cashews.
-beef curry with coconut milk.

"OH MY GOD I WILL GET BORED!"

This is what most people say originally.

First, to spice things up, go to the herbs and spices section and get as many of those as you want. You can go all Gordon Ramsey and add as many herbs and spices as you like. This alone gives you around 15 different ways you can just make chicken taste!

Download our FREE Recipes: 365performance.com.au/book.

But before we move on, I just want you to stop and ask yourself – "is it true?" Is it true you don't like eating the same thing? I see lots of people come to us and that's the first thing that comes out of their mouth when we mention eating healthy. It isn't true that they have to eat the same thing, or that the food is boring – with our recipes and ideas below the food is always different and tastes amazing…

But most people have this overriding story that they can't eat the same thing all the time.

The funny thing is, those same people normally have nachos every second day, or ate coco pops or vegemite toast for 18 years of their life every morning, or drink the same beer every night…

It all starts upstairs in your mind. What are the stories that you tell yourself?

Eat for POWER and ENERGY and LIFE not just for TASTE!

TAKEAWAY OPTIONS:
Oporto's - get a chicken salad.
Supermarket - get a roast chicken, or tin of salmon with some blueberries and some nuts.
McDonald's - get one of their salads.
Subway - as above.

"Oh my god I can't get a salad from McDonald's" – yes you can. Same deal as before, is it the most perfect option? Probably not. But it is a lot better than getting a double quarter pounder with large fries and large coke.

THE CHEAT MEAL:
I don't like the idea of calling it a cheat. I call it being human. If you follow this way that we propose, it will get to a point that the last thing you would actually want is a huge pizza and a bunch of rubbish because you know how it will make you feel after – tired, bloated, sluggish...

But if you do have it or want it, just make sure you do your best to not do it very often. Once a week is a good gap between these types of meals initially.

One thing I do want to talk about though is the cheat meal weigh in.

So many people eat well, get on the scales every day (even though they shouldn't), and begin to see progress.

Then they have a cheat meal on a Saturday night and step on the scales the following morning and see that they have put on 2-3kg and want to give up.

Here's the thing.

You don't put on 3kg of FAT overnight from a cheat meal.

You put on 3kg of water.

When you are eating clean – a balanced diet with protein, fat, and veg and limiting all those starches like bread etc. Your body doesn't retain water as much...

But when you have things like a pizza, or maybe a big serving of cake or pasta, these foods do.

So, it's important to not let the scales get to you the next day.

After your meal where you enjoyed yourself, wake up the next day, maybe go for a walk to burn off some of those extra calories, go back to eating clean and by the next day you will be back to where you were before that meal.

As you begin to move more and eat better, your body will begin to change.

Do not let the scales be the thing you go by.

It really isn't rocket science.

If you eat well and move more the weight drops.

If you eat poor and move less the weight increases.

It is important especially as your training increases, to get measurements done (we do this for all of our members) and monitor body fat changing.

Many of our clients can have their weight stay the same for a month, but their pants size drops and their body fat goes down 5-10%!

NEXT STEPS:
Clean out the fridge and pantry – get rid of all the rubbish! The soft drink, the treats, the food with no nutritional value.

Donate the food to a homeless shelter or somewhere that it can be used – it doesn't serve you!

Download our FREE Recipes: 365performance.com.au/book.

Go shopping for all the healthy items we discussed above… And cook!

Remember, you don't need to eat 100% perfect 100% of the time!

If you do that, you will have success for a week or two and then bail completely because you can't cope.

Instead, aim for PROGRESS not PERFECTION.

And you will get there.

9 MOVE

"If you are in a bad mood go for a walk.
If you are still in a bad mood go for another walk."
— Hippocrates

Sweating is not the secret to your salvation.

It starts with the mind first.

Your nutrition second.

Moving is the icing on the cake.

…Why?

First, it is the exact opposite to the way 90% of the population do things, so already we should know we are on the right track!

But I will elaborate.

Firstly, if your mind isn't clear and you are letting people and events trigger you, you will constantly end up going to that 'place'. That place we discussed earlier where you either over eat, or eat rubbish, or drink heaps of alcohol, or choose to not do anything but sit on your bum and watch TV for 6 hours. In these times of frustration and anger, you are automatically going to be eating more calories than you require and moving less, which will cause weight gain.

Secondly, if your nutrition isn't dialed in, then on a daily basis you will be malnourished and in most cases eating excess calories. This will not only cause weight gain, but also limit your ability to recover and your bodies adaptation to any of the moving that you do – making it essentially a waste of time!

Most people don't address the above two pieces, and simply start training.

By training they will on average burn around 300 calories based off of their intensity level as a beginner.

Which is the equivalent of a donut.

So they are literally beginning training to burn off the top end of some bad choices they make. They may not put on more weight, but they don't begin to lose any either.

I will say that again, and please understand it. Most people eat more calories than they require and subsequently put on weight. By not addressing this and simply training, all they are doing is 'burning off' those excess calories. They are still eating too much, so by training all they are doing is off-setting their excess calorie consumption.

In the past (without training) they may stand on the scales on the first of the month and by the end of the month they are up one kilogram. So they recognise this and they try to be healthier so they start training. The next month on the first they stand on their scales again and this time begin training. By training they have burnt off those excess calories they consumed during the month. They then stand on the scales at the end of the month, the scales are not up one kilogram like in the past (which is progress that they don't recognise), but their weight is exactly the same. Due to them only off-setting their bad habits.

The path to achieving success is to focus your time and energy on doing the work to help with your mindset first and to work on your nutrition second. Only by doing this will you begin to fuel your body with the adequate nutrition it needs on a consistent basis to avoid being in a caloric surplus and get you the results you want.

Body composition changes will already begin simply from the change in mindset coupled with the nutrition focus as discussed above.

Once again – The moving is the icing on the cake.

I see many people who might have a busy few days, they haven't done their meal prep, but don't want to miss out their training session.

So they go for their 30 min walk or go to the gym.

They miss out on meal prepping.

And spend the next 3 days having a rubbish lunch due to not taking their own lunch to work, and consuming an extra 1,000 calories than normal.

It sounds silly, but it is important to remember.

Training and moving your body should only happen once you have set yourself up for success with your nutrition.

Yes, I know I am repeating myself.

I have had many clients who would train with me only once a week and then work on their nutrition and lose 1kg consistently a week.

I have had many other clients who come to us who would train 5x/week in the past, not work on their nutrition or headspace at all, and never got results — success leaves clues!

But once you have got it sorted. What should you do?

Do you remember the main principle?

Move a bit more – relative to how much you are moving at the moment.

BUT! BUT! BUT! BUT! How often? For how long? How hard? What do I do?

…The chaos of complexity is back!

Don't stress. Just do a bit more than you normally do.

I have met people who have literally done NOTHING for 25 years.

They start with us and think if they don't train 5 days per week they are a failure.

If they trained ONCE a WEEK they are already 500000% improved from who they were previously!

Remember, PROGRESS not PERFECTION.

But, to give you some guidelines...

What should you do?

Most people will come in or call us up, wanting to make a change but then say something like "I am not fit enough to start".

That is the equivalent of saying you want to run a 5k, but you aren't fit enough to do that yet, so you are going to start swimming to get fitter before you start training for the 5k.

If you want to run a 5k, you start running... Maybe 100m, maybe 1,000m... But you start running.

So my first question isn't to tell you what you SHOULD do, my question is to ask you what you WANT to do? What would you LIKE to do?

This is where the first conflict lies. As people think they NEED to do a certain type of training to get results.

Do you WANT to be training on your own, have no support, and just do your own thing? Maybe you might want to start walking, running, swimming, going to a regular gym.

Do you WANT to be training with other people who are on the same journey as you, have constant support and coaching from qualified people, be held accountable, and ensure you are doing everything correct to get to your targets? Maybe you might want to reach out to us (shameless plug).

I obviously have my bias. After doing different types of training all my life, We have found and created what I believe to be the absolute best choice for BALANCED health and fitness.

But at the end of the day I don't care what you do, just MOVE.

How often?

This is a tough one to answer in a book as I don't know you as an individual and your previous experience and history...

But look back from your past.

Are you that girl who goes all-out right from the beginning, pushes through the resistance at the start and does something every day and then falls in love with it?

Or are you that guy who goes all-out right from the beginning, does too much too soon and can't cope, and then after 2 weeks you stop and give up?

For some it may be easier to go for a 20 min walk every single day first thing when they wake up or at lunch every day.

For others, it may be better to train with us personally every Monday, Tuesday, Thursday and Friday.

For others, it may be better to go for a swim Monday, rest Tuesday, long walk Wednesday, personal training Thursday, rest Friday, and a long walk Saturday and Sunday.

What I am saying? Do whatever you want.

Move a bit more – relative to how much you are moving at the moment.

How long?

Hopefully the above has already given you some insight as to what I am going to say here...

But for most people, same deal.

You want to make this work relative to what you can handle.

For me and some others, I personally LOVE to go for a 1 hour walk, with my podcast playing, to just clear my head.

Three to four times a week I train with our clients doing a class.

There are other times when I am time poor and I am better suited to do something short. Many mornings I will wake up first thing and just go for a 10-min jog.

SOMETHING is better than NOTHING.

Move a bit more – relative to how much you are moving at the moment

How hard?

This is one you want to stop and think about for a moment.

Harder hurts more.

I remember one day I really couldn't be bothered training (this happens all the time by the way!). I was meant to go for a run, I was training for a marathon and was meant to run for around an hour. I knew how far I went last time, and I wanted to try and beat that distance. But in my head, I knew if I set out to try and beat that distance, I would have had to run faster, and it would have hurt more…

Knowing that, I almost decided to not go for the run.

Instead, I stopped for a moment and thought about what I am grateful for with my body – grateful for my ability to run pain free, grateful to be able to have the choice to go outside in that moment and be in the sun in the park, grateful to be able to be free of the back pain I suffered for all those years…

Feeling a little flat, I decided to just run, and not care how far I went. To run a bit slower than normal… and just run and be free of any stress of doing a better time or anything like that.

I laced up my shoes and started running. By 10 min in I felt terrific. I went around 5% easier than normal but the actual run was 10x more enjoyable. I was looking around more, taking everything in, not hurting as much…

And when I finished, I felt so much more alive. So happy I didn't give in and pushed through that other voice on my shoulder that comes up and wants to hold me back…

Moral of the story: There is nobody who finishes a training session and looks back and says, 'I wish I slept in and didn't do that'. It might be tough to get moving, and not every day should be your BEST day. Just every day move. Some days go harder, some days go easier, but every day move.

BONUS: The invisible exerciser

We are inherently tough on ourselves.

We recognise when we move more.

We recognise when we eat our healthy lunch.

But we always fail to recognise when we are focused and saying NO to those things that have held us back all those years.

When we say NO to the lunchtime cake at work.
When we say NO to the after-work drinks.
When we say NO to the box of donuts at the family lunch.
When we say NO to the large mocha frappe at breakfast.

But all these things add up. Simply having one of the choices above would require a whole training session in most cases to burn off. Depending on how much you used to go to town on yourself, it may be 2-3 sessions.

But it's extremely important that we identify these situations when they pop up, and recognise how 'old you' would have said YES – and 'new you' just said NO...

It helps give you even more momentum and motivation.

By saying NO to that lunchtime cake at work when you normally would have, your training session isn't to work that bad decision off, as you aren't in a caloric surplus from making that poor choice... Instead, the training you are going to do is going to help you get even closer to your goals.

Always recognise the power of a NO when you make that choice.

It can be tough at times.

But not as tough as saying yes and having to deal with the consequences of it after!

The best choice?

For those who don't want to go at it alone…

When it comes to mindset, training and nutrition I firmly believe that nothing comes close to what we offer at 365 Performance.

Compared to a regular gym where you walk in and nobody talks to you and knows your name… Where everyone is self-conscious and there are mirrors everywhere… Where you get no guidance and support at all…

Or other fitness 'classes' where you walk in and simply get yelled at or paying a coach to count reps and learn technique from a computer screen… Or where you don't really know what you are doing and simply copy the person next to you – who doesn't know what they are doing either!

What we have is different.

All of our coaches were once a client of mine. They all have different backgrounds, challenges and experiences they have had to overcome to arrive where they are today. Having such great variety of coaches allow every single one of them to resonate with different client's relative to where they are at.

Our coaches work with you intimately. Not just during the sessions by giving you personalised coaching, but also outside of the sessions by offering personalised nutrition and lifestyle advice. As well as constant check-in's and measurements to ensure you are seeing success.

All in an environment that is completely ego and intimidation free.

The best part – before anyone starts with us we take them through a thorough assessment to ensure they don't have any underlying issues or injuries, and anything that is there we put a plan in place to work with and actively fix so you don't get injured or hurt yourself. And most importantly, we teach you all the movements in a private setting so before you start doing the regular sessions with us you already have the confidence on how to move correctly and know what you are doing, so you are set up for success from day one.

Tegan Wotton reviewed 365 Performance – ⑤★
28 June at 14:35 · 🌐

I've always trained in some capacity or another, but since joining 365 Performance my strength, overall fitness and physique has improved. On top of this, I have learnt so much about my body as well as its capabilities and completely revamped my thinking (in a positive way!) to nutrition and exercise. This is a credit to the coaches at 365 Performance who promote a holistic approach to wellness which encompasses education, nutrition, healthy habits and of course, lifting weights.

Alexander Song reviewed 365 Performance – ⑤★
12 October 2016 · 🌐

Awesome experienced coaches who are dedicated to help you with personal goals in fitness either be in nutrition or exercise. The exercises are different everyday so it's never a dull moment making it fun!!! The place has a great feel to it with great people and you can be at any level of fitness to start. Highly recommended!!!

Mick Wasabi reviewed 365 Performance – ⑤★
17 hrs · 🌐

My wife and I have been members of 365 Performance for over a year now and have both loved every second of it. We've been to a fair few crossfit gyms all over the world and have had mixed experiences with them. But not one of them can compete with 365. The staff have become our extended family with their extremely approachable personalities. The gym is always clean and tidy, and the workouts are always fun and rewarding (after its finished). I recommend this place to anyone looking at all round fitness and health gains. Whether you're just starting out or you're looking for a challenge, they will discover your needs, discuss your goals and help you achieve every single one of them. If you want a better quality of life, 365 is where it's at.

Dave Duke reviewed 365 Performance – ⑤★
28 June at 20:03 · 🌐

Doesn't matter what age, fitness, health or skill level you are 365 Performance is the place to train and get better. Awesome & professional Coaches, great facilities, great programs and I wouldn't think of training anywhere else. They changed my life for the better, great work 365 Performance!

Lena Petelo reviewed 365 Performance – 5★
18 July 2016 ·

You can't get this kind of experience anywhere else. This community is special. The coaches are exceptional and the members are wonderful, down to earth and amazingly inspiring. Highly recommend this gym to those who want to be part of something special. We are big, small, tall, short, black and white! Ego friendly and very family orientated.
Come meet our amazing coaches and members and be part of our 365 family 🖤

David Horsnell reviewed 365 Performance – 5★
3 July at 19:02 ·

I hadn't trained or played any sport in over 15 years I was unhealthy and overweight and I can honestly say I am physically and mentally in the best shape of my life.
It took me a while to build up the courage to walk in to 365 performance but once I did everyone was so friendly and positive I soon found myself looking forward to training it's my favourite part of the day.
365 performance has help me in my life so much more than just loosing a few kilos I highly recommend anyone who wants to join to just do it you won't regret it.

Nathan Osborne reviewed 365 Performance – 5★
22 September 2016 ·

365 Performance is by far the best Gym experience I've ever had. Professional, supportive and most importantly they make it enjoyable. You want to turn up and look forward to going to daily sessions. The Coaches at 365 go above and beyond whilst your at the gym and even when you are not, regularly contacting you to add that personal touch by checking your progress and how you are feeling. As the motto says "More than Fitness", 365 Performance not only help you with a work out but they support you with your lifestyle, mobility and nutrition education. Call or drop in today, you won't regret it!

Heather Palmer Laybutt reviewed 365 Performance – 5★
20 July 2016 ·

I really feel part of the community so I actually look forward to going to the gym to catch up with the people. Everyone is welcome!

Julie Hastings reviewed 365 Performance – ⭐
18 July 2016 ·

I love training here. It is definitely more than just fitness, I walked in with fitness goals after having my second child and now have many more personal and professional goals because of the inspiration. Highly recommend. Great support, excellent coaches and a community that oozes spirit and soul.

Graham Laybutt reviewed 365 Performance – ⭐
19 July 2016 ·

More than fitness!
Come down and check out 365 Performance.
Professional, knowledgeable coaches who LISTEN to you and actually care about you and your goals.
Our community is second to none: Fun, Friends, FAMILY!
What are you waiting for?
Come down and check us out!!

Katherine Jones reviewed CrossFit Chipping Norton – ⭐
5 July at 21:39 ·

There were so many things that prevented me from joining 365 sooner than I did. I was convinced I wasn't strong enough/fit enough/ capable of joining in and I was so nervous about walking in on the first night. I soon became aware that 365 is not just a gym, it's a community full of amazing and supportive people that want to see you do your best- no matter your experience or skill level. The staff here are the most down to earth and supportive coaches I've ever met, not to mention so knowledgable. Whatever your goal and whatever your capability the coaches tailor the work out to you. In 9 weeks I've lost a total of 17cm and I've never felt better or stronger. If this is something you're considering, I can't encourage you enough to take the plunge and have a go. You will be welcomed by every person you meet, you'll have an amazing new group of people to call your friends, and you'll soon wonder what you ever did before 365!!

Chantal Munro reviewed CrossFit Chipping Norton – ⭐
28 September 2016 ·

'More than fitness' is their motto and this is 100% the truth! They obviously care about fitness but more importantly they care about each individual and their wellbeing. From saying hi when you walk in, to keeping track of measurements, to meal plans and nutrition advice, this is by far the best gym Ive attended!

Graham Wilson reviewed CrossFit Chipping Norton – 5★
31 October 2016 ·

I have been doing PT at CrossFit for over two years now. The expert coaches have made a huge difference to my mobility, strength and fitness. I highly recommend Scott and his coaches at this gym.

Angela Ebid reviewed CrossFit Chipping Norton – 5★
19 July at 21:02 ·

Really lives up to the motto "more than fitness". It's definitely a space of growth and resilience. The coaches are highly skilled and cater for each individual's fitness level. Such a caring and motivating community, absolutely blessed to be a part of it all.

Belinda Searle reviewed CrossFit Chipping Norton – 5★
30 September 2016 ·

I have never been to a gym where I have received so much support from the coaches.
I receive a fortnightly email from my mentor just to check how I'm going with training.
Training is fun & the atmosphere is friendly.
I have achieved some amazing results since I joined 1 year ago all due to the encouragement of the coaches.

Larnie Elana Valley reviewed CrossFit Milperra – 5★
3 November 2016 ·

This place is like no other.. fun, friends, family, fitness, future! My biggest regret is not joining sooner... Their holistic approach to fitness and attention to detail regarding physical, mental and social health is second-to-none...

John Stambouli reviewed CrossFit Milperra – 5★
29 June at 14:47 ·

There is something special about this place , The training is fantastic and caters for all levels and people but the magic isn't in the training (even though I love the programming) ..Its in the COMMUNITY.. This is what makes the place truly special..You feel at home right away and bond with people who quickly go from gym partners to friends to FAMILY.. I like to think of it as my second home !
If you are looking to be a serious athlete, to lose a little weight or just meet some like minded people whilst you get a sweat on then there is no better place !

The only regret I have is I didnt SIGN UP EARLIER !

Love it and wouldn't train anywhere else !

10 WHAT NOW?

This book exists only to help create a possibility in your mind.

A possibility for you to get what you really want.

And to hopefully allow you to give yourself the permission to achieve it.

There will be hurdles.

There will be obstacles to overcome.

As humans, we are brought up that it is a sign of weakness to ask for help, to get supported...

But in most cases, when it comes to health and fitness, people think they can simply join a gym and eat some chicken breast and broccoli and that's it. If it was that easy we would all be walking around looking like a Victoria's Secret model in 2 months.

When it comes down to it, that would be the equivalent of you thinking I could do YOUR job for a week, with no training... You would come back to work and be wondering why the place is burning down.

It's the same deal... I wouldn't have success with your job because I wouldn't have had the experience and coaching necessary to know how to do it properly.

With your health, it is exactly the same.

Far too many of us go at it alone.

I want to say that the only sign of weakness IS going at it alone.

Not being open to help.

Telling yourself that you have 'GOT THIS' – when clearly you don't.

It is the best investment you can make. You already know how much improving your health and fitness will benefit those around you and every area of your life. Don't discount it and spend less money on your health per week than you would on beer or coffee. **You are worth it. Your family is worth it.**

Sometimes the only missing thing to your success is an environment free of intimidation…

For others, it is being around a community that support you and lift you up – not bring you down…

For others, it may just be a conversation…

For others, it is accountability…

For others, it is support…

For others, it is nothing else but some guidance on their nutrition, or a push with their training…

But at the end of the day, at times we must simply let go in order to grow, and not do everything on our own.

When you have a team around you to support and lead you through the tough times when they come up, success is a lot easier to achieve.

Hopefully this book has allowed you to not only understand yourself a little better and guide you to achieve more, but to also recognise that my team and I are just regular people like you who overcame our own challenges.

If we have resonated with you, and providing we aren't booked out at the moment, we would love to be able to sit down and see if we are a good fit.

If you are interested in making a change and working with us, go to 365performance.com.au and fill out a consult request.

If you haven't already, make sure you subscribe to our Podcast. Simply search for 'The 365 Performance Show' on iTunes, Google Play, or Stitcher. Alternatively go to **365performance.com.au/podcast**.

Make sure you access the bonuses for this book at **365performance.com.au/book**.

And finally, if this book has been of benefit to you in some way, please let others know about it so you can make an impact on their lives and help them Stop Stopping. You can also order them a copy using the link above.

I am so grateful you have taken time out of your life to read this.

To your health.

Scott Dillon.

ACKNOWLEDGEMENTS

To all of my mentors and people I have learnt from up until this moment and into the future. But specifically, people that created moments of awareness that liberated me from my prison and gave me the tools to do the same with others. Byron Katie, Dr. John Demartini, James FitzGerald, Sharon Prete, Mark Twight, Dan Millman, Tony Robins, Garret J White.

To all of our clients, past and present, thank you for trusting in us. After years and years of tears, mistakes, learning, struggles and growth, I wouldn't have life any other way. You are why my staff and I get up in the morning and we count every day as a gift that we are able to lead and serve you in a small way.

To my staff – past and present, thank you for standing by my side, leading with me, and teaching me more than you could ever know.

To my mate Steven Marrs who left us, thank you for giving me a tiny opportunity that allowed me to take a leap in this world to make a difference, I hope you are free of pain now and can look down and see the impact we are having.

To my parents. You created this.

To Aroha. For arriving by my side in the darkness, I love you and owe you my life.